FEEL 20!

Hormone Replacement and Nutrient Solutions

For Better:

Energy,
    Mood,
        Sleep
            Weight,
                Health
                    Sex & Intimacy

Your Friends Will Beg To Find Out What You Did!

Paul Thomas, M.D.

TABLE OF CONTENTS

ACKNOWLEDGMENTS

I owe most of my knowledge and wisdom to my patients and their families. Those who have suffered the most through the years have so often pushed me to dig deeper for answers and explanations.

My patient, whom I call "Joe" in this book, was particularly instrumental in inspiring further research on the connection between the hormone testosterone and the symptoms of anxiety and depersonalization. Since this is a relatively new area of knowledge, there will be ongoing studies both in support of and against this connection. It is without question, however, that in certain patients the link is powerful and debilitating. Thankfully the symptoms are reversible with the optimization of hormones.

In my quest to learn as much as possible about hormones and in particular the use of bio-identical hormones, my gratitude goes to Dr Neil Rouser. His book, How to Achieve Healthy Aging and his trainings offered to professionals, were vital. He is a pioneer and has the courage and willingness to share his knowledge and understanding for the good of all.

I owe a special thanks to Lef Hylton, Winnie Thomas and Erica Zelfand ND, for assistance in reading, encouragement and suggestions. I owe my wife Maiya gratitude for ongoing support and encouragement that enables me to work too hard, study, and take the time to write and research and tackle new projects. She says as long as she sees the twinkle in my eye and my excitement about what I am doing, she is behind me, even if it means sacrificing her own time with me. I'm blessed with supportive family and children who all encourage and support me.

FOREWORD

Are you tired of being sick and tired? Have you had doctor after doctor seem not to care, not to listen, or not to understand? Have you been told you are "just depressed", or it's anxiety or "you are fine", that there is nothing physically wrong with you, but you know there is something just not right? Have you been told your bloodwork is normal but you know something is wrong? Are you tired all of the time, anxious or depressed, having trouble getting good sleep and waking up rested and full of energy and excitement for the day? Are you thinking that your weight gain, fatigue, muscles aches, headaches, mood swings, lack of libido, and many other health issues are just the way it's going to be?

Thankfully there is a solution. You may be experiencing symptoms of hormone and nutrient deficiencies. You may have food sensitivities, or even be overloaded with toxins. By addressing these four areas with specific testing and treatment recommendations, the healthy life of your dreams is just months away.

Are you aware that your environment, the food you eat, what you drink, and the air you breathe, may be robbing you of health and vitality? Do you know that you are absolutely missing some key nutrients that you need? Are you aware that certain foods are creating an immune response that keeps you feeling tired, foggy, and ill? Do you think that you may have some habits or behaviors that are sabotaging your health?

This book will provide you with answers to all of these questions.

As a physician, board certified in Integrative Holistic Medicine, Pediatrics, and Addiction Medicine, I bring a unique perspective and refreshingly simple approach to reclaiming your health. I have helped numerous persons regain vitality, mental function, and a level of wellness that simply didn't exist before, despite countless other doctor and specialist visits and approaches.

Your benefits from reading and implementing the simple ideas in this book include:
- Increased energy
- Improved sleep
- Less anxiety and depression
- Better sexual function and intimacy
- Optimal weight
- Improved health and wellness
- Reduced dependence on medications
- Increased strength and fitness

Evidence supporting the efficacy of hormone replacement therapy and nutritional supplementation is abundant for those willing to look beyond the hopeless message of the pharmaceutical industry. Countless post-menopausal women are saying "I'm having the best sex ever," and men both young and old alike are regaining function, muscle, and strength, while losing the anxiety and depression that in so many was virtually incapacitating them.

If you read this book, and implement a handful of suggestions within, you will become the master of your own health destiny. You will experience a new level of energy and joy of living. You will learn the best-kept secrets of the health industry, unknown to most traditional doctors and experts. You will need to read this book to fulfill your destiny of health and wellness. You can live the lifestyle you really want. Imagine how you will feel to wake up with energy, rested and ready to get moving. Imagine your friends and loved ones asking you, "What the heck you are doing, you look so healthy and energetic?"

For the person living with a hormonal deficiency, replacing hormones using natural biologically identical hormones has health and well-being benefits that cannot be achieved in any other way. This book will help you understand why you have hormone deficiencies, nutrient deficiencies, food sensitivities, and a build-up of toxins keeping you ill with compromised energy and vitality.

You will learn exactly what to do, which tests to get (just a few will give you the road map back to health), where to go to get these tests done, and exactly how to replace your deficiencies and get back your health, energy, vitality, libido, and general wellbeing.

Are you ready to dive into the book? In less than two hours you will have the keys to amazing health, energy, fitness, and all the fringe benefits that come from optimal health. Start your journey and turn the page.

INTRODUCTION: True stories

There's a story I need to tell you so you will understand how I stumbled on the truths revealed in this book that are largely unknown or ignored. When you discover something this big, you just must tell the world about it, and hence this book is my testimony and proof to you that this works. Names have been changed to protect the identity of the individuals.

JOE

Two years ago, "Joe," a 26 year old, young man, was struggling with an addiction to alcohol. He was given a shot of Vivitrol (a medication sometimes used to block the pleasurable effects of alcohol and opiates). Within two hours, he was thrown into the worst depression that I have ever witnessed in my 25 years as a doctor. He had never before been clinically depressed. He immediately became so anxious, depressed, and depersonalized that he could no longer work his job. He had to move back in with his parents and could not leave the house. He was even hospitalized for severe suicidal thoughts. His psychiatrist tried every medicine known but with no positive results. He even went through months of RTMS (Repetitive Transcranial Magnetic Stimulation), with little relief from his dark state. His depression, depersonalization and inability to work lasted for more than a year;
While researching on the Internet, "Joe" stumbled on the fact that his symptoms of depersonalization, anxiety, and depression matched the symptoms of low testosterone.

Joe asked his psychiatrist to order testosterone levels, which he did. To everyone's surprise, Joe had a total testosterone level below 200 and a free testosterone level below 50. (Normal levels for his age, were 380-1200 total testosterone and 80-240 free testosterone).

He was referred to his primary care doctor, who had only occasionally treated old men with testosterone and was reluctant to treat Joe, but ultimately agreed. Within a month Joe was feeling better than he had for over a year. He moved back in with his girlfriend and was able to go back to work.

Men In Detox

In addition to my primary care clinic, I run an office-based detox program to help young adults and teenagers get off of opiates like heroin, methadone, and pain pills. I noticed that most of my addiction and opioid-dependent patients were extremely anxious. This was a symptom I had previously attributed to their addictions and never considered that there may be a hormonal deficiency responsible for these symptoms. Virtually every young man with anxiety in my addiction clinic when tested, had low testosterone. When placed on testosterone replacement therapy, their energy improved, their anxiety was significantly reduced, and for the many who had either lost interest in sex, or in some cases were unable to maintain an erection, these challenges disappeared.

EVE

"Eve" was in her late 50's, and had been through a hysterectomy-oophorectomy (removal of uterus and ovaries) in her 40's. She had been on synthetic hormone replacement (birth-control pills) since that time. When the WHI study published risks of hormone replacement, she went off of the hormones for a while but suffered severe menopause symptoms, with hot flashes, weight gain, and fatigue. Ultimately, Eve went back on the hormones. After evaluating her nutrient and hormone levels, I prescribed bio-identical hormones (estradiol, progesterone, testosterone, DHEA, and armour thyroid), and the appropriate nutritional supplements. Her fatigue disappeared and she dropped 20 pounds in 6 months.

ADAM

Eve's husband "Adam" was fortunate enough to have had his hormones and nutrients tested and treated at the same time as his wife. In his mid 50's, he had a BMI of 30, weighed 225 pounds, and had lost interest in sex. He could not lose weight and frequent injuries seemed to persist preventing him from exercising. If he could exercise, the fatigue he felt kept him from doing anything other than surviving the workday and collapsing on the Lazy Boy. Testing showed he was severely low in vitamin D and B12. Testosterone and DHEA (a testosterone precursor) were low for his age and his TSH was high, indicating low thyroid function. With nutrient and hormone optimization, Adam now weighs less than 200 pounds for the first time in decades. He has energy to spare and feels 20, with early morning erections and the desire and endurance to keep up with Eve's new found desires and energy.

Teen Patients

Seeing that countless patients in my addiction clinic all seemed to have anxiety and fatigue, I wondered if perhaps the teenagers with similar symptoms in my pediatric clinic might likewise have low testosterone, as well as hormone and nutrient imbalances. I have now discovered many teenage boys (past puberty) who have testosterone levels of an eighty-year old man. Vitamin D deficiency is almost universal, and patients of any age typically will have several nutrient deficiencies.

ANN

A client new to my practice, "Ann", was an infant, of nine months. She had been having daily seizures for several months. She had very poor tone, and no control of her eye movements. She had been seen by several child neurologists in town, and had been tried on virtually every anti-seizure medication. Micronutrient testing showed severe lack of B-12 in her cells. Methyl-B-12 shots twice a week had her seizure-free, eyes normal, and tone virtually normal within a month.

If you have any chronic condition, you owe it to yourself to get micronutrient testing and a thorough hormone evaluation. In order to get the most health benefits from the optimization of your nutrients and hormones, there are a few other areas of health you need to address. This will help you to build a solid health foundation, and is the topic of the next chapter. You won't want to miss this vital information and get your journey to optimal energy, health, and wellbeing started.

Health, Fitness, and Wellness
The Foundation

Imagine being a generally fit child and teenager, with few health concerns other than occasional childhood colds, ear infections, or strep throat. If you are a child of the past 20 years, you add allergies, eczema, asthma, developmental and psychiatric issues (from anxiety and depression to ADD, ADHD, Autism Spectrum Disorder, as well as all the various language and learning challenges that are more prevalent the past 10–20 years).

Now fast forward to age 25 or 30. You likely have trouble sleeping, your energy is low, and you may struggle with addictions. Perhaps you struggle with energy or getting enough quality sleep without the help of prescriptions, drugs, and/or alcohol. What happened to that carefree joy of life you had as a kid?

By age 40–50, you are definitely struggling to get quality sleep. You are tired all the time, run down, and may be struggling with your weight gain. Perhaps you've tried multiple "diets." If you don't have diabetes or high blood pressure, you may be pre-diabetic such that you get weak and shaky if you don't eat often or if you eat a high carbohydrate meal. You have developed insulin resistance, so carbohydrates are just stored as fat even if you are relatively careful with how much you are eating.

After age 50, in addition to all of the above, you may be struggling with increased fatigue, poor sex drive, low energy, and poor sleep. You may be on more than one prescription drug as doctors get busy treating the various symptoms related to your deteriorating health. If you were unable to conquer any addictions you may have acquired along the way, they are now killing you.

THERE IS A SOLUTION. You can rebuild your health and wellbeing. If you are ready to take that journey and reclaim the health of your childhood (minus the childhood illnesses), this chapter will outline the key steps necessary to return you to a vibrant youth-like zest for life with a body to match that energy and zest.

If you are reading this book, you are most likely interested in the benefits that bio-identical hormone replacement can provide you. I can assure you the benefits are tremendous and a key part of regaining your youthful energy, libido, and vibrant health if you have hormone deficiencies. You will not, however, enjoy that total package of appropriate weight, muscle development, reversal of insulin sensitivity, and the exchange of fatigue with youthful energy if you do not address the issues in this chapter.

Diet

We are what we eat. I remember hearing this long ago and just blowing it off with the thought "yeah right." As far back as Aristotle's "Food is your medicine," there has been the knowledge of the direct link between what we eat and our health. It actually makes complete sense. Every bit of our body is made up of molecules that are built from what? The food our mom's ate when we were in the womb, and then the food we eat after we are born, period!

Avoid all GMO (Genetically Modified Organism) foods. You are going to have to make some sacrifices to get this diet issue right. We cannot rebuild health if we continue to poison ourselves. Genetically modified foods have been banned in about 30 countries, including all of Europe. The scientists in these countries have concluded that the dangers are real and extremely detrimental to the health of people and livestock. If you live in the USA, you are part of the largest experiment on a population ever conducted, and it's not going well.

You may suffer from allergies, eczema, asthma, autoimmune disorders (Hashimoto's Thyroiditis, diabetes, arthritis, MS, and so on) and the neuropsychiatric disorders, all of which may in part be triggered by the toxicity of GMO foods. So what does that mean? You cannot, in the USA, eat soy or corn or anything sweet unless it is labeled as organic or GMO-free. We do not yet have GMO label-laws, as the industry has, so far, been able to defeat the laws to require this labeling. Do you think if your food (anything in a bag or box) had a skull and crossbones on it you would buy it? 90% of corn and soy in the USA has GMO and these products are in virtually all store-bought or fast food products.

The next step in your diet is to eat organic. You should not consume pesticides with their known toxicity. If you cannot afford to do this, then at least be very thorough in your washing of the produce and learn which foods are particularly high in pesticides. The environmental working group (EWG) is a great resource for this.

Drink filtered water. If at all possible, you want the water to pass through a charcoal filter. If you have reverse osmosis as well, that is even better. Water in most USA cities is very contaminated with pesticides and herbicides far above known safe levels.

So all I've asked is that you eat organic (no GMO) foods and drink good water. With effort, you can do this. The next and probably the most important step is what you eat. Most of us do not do well with gluten, the protein in wheat, barley, rye and spelt. If you need proof of this, we can order a food sensitivity panel that looks at your IgG against about 100 different foods. If you show a huge reaction (high IgG) then your body is trying to attack this food as if it were an invader, much like we do against chicken pox, measles, strep throat, and other infections. Removing those foods that are triggering an immune response will start the journey of healing.

The second most important health aspect to your diet is that it be real food (plant and animals in their natural state). The industrial age brought with it highly processed food. Highly refined flour and sugar (along with substitutes) are the enemy of our health. These put our system in a state of stress. Our bodies must make a lot of insulin to keep our blood sugar stable. In the process, we store more fat, and eventually our cells become resistant to the insulin. You have now entered that wonderful world of easy weight gain no matter what you seem to do.

Thankfully, if you keep your insulin low, you can lose weight and regain your health. So what can we eat?

All the vegetables we want! Eat lean meats. For those grains to which we don't have sensitivities, we should eat them in as whole of a state as possible. Better to eat steel cut oats instead of whole rolled, and never eat the quick oats that are even more refined. Eat brown rice instead of the nutrient-poor white rice. If you can tolerate gluten, then eat whole grains in moderation.

There are numerous diet books out there. All of those that promote healthy and sustained weight loss share the feature of reducing processed carbohydrates. If they don't, then they are simply starvation diets that you won't be able to sustain and your energy level will suffer.

If you have special circumstances, such as autism, inflammatory bowel disease, or other gastrointestinal challenges that make the above advice impractical or impossible, then by all means consult your physician, and consider the GAPS diet.

Absolutely no soda! High fructose corn syrup is not only GMO but it is death to the pancreas, leading directly to insulin resistance and weight gain, fatigue, and a host of health problems. The sugar in regular soda (if it's sugar at all) is GMO. Aspartame, in diet soda in this country, gets converted to formaldehyde in our bodies – a literal poison. I'm embarrassed to tell you I was a big diet coke fan until I learned the truth about aspartame in Woodrow Monte's book While Science Sleeps.

Water (filtered) is the drink of choice. Drink lots of water. An adult should have at least 6–8 glasses a day. Aim for a gallon (3000 ml for men and 2200ml for women). For variety, add a twist of lemon, lime or orange. Make some natural organic tea, or even coffee. The caffeine in most teas and coffee is a problem if you are taking over 200 mg of caffeine a day.
500 mg of caffeine can cause heart arrhythmias and has been known to cause death. I still drink coffee (not many vices left)! Energy drinks and other commercial drinks have problems, like artificial colors and flavors, and generally too much caffeine.

Alcoholic beverages are tricky. If you have been drinking daily you should consider getting help, and get all alcohol out of your life. There are studies showing that a small glass of red wine, and now some studies even showing that a small amount of white wine, may have health benefits. If you truly can take it or leave it, and you are of drinking age and you can stop at that half a glass (6 ounces) limit per day, you may be someone who has no propensity to become addicted or develop tolerance. If this is your situation, the occasional small intake of alcohol may actually provide you with health benefits. I still think it may be risky if you do this on a daily basis, especially if you get intoxicated in any way or feel neurological effects from the drink.

VITAMINS & SUPPLEMENTS

You may have heard that you can get all your nutrients from your diet if you eat a well-rounded diet. I think that is close to the truth, but in practical terms not possible. Micronutrient testing in my practice has shown that fewer than 1% of us have optimal levels of all the key nutrients. Spectracell offers a patented unique assay of nutrient function in the live cell (lymphocyte) that will show in many cases that even where serum levels are adequate the functional level inside the cell may not be adequate.

Vitamin D

Unless you are a lifeguard near the equator who has their shirt off much of the day, you are most likely not getting adequate sun exposure to make enough Vitamin D. I have tested over 1000 patients and not one had an optimal Vitamin D level. The levels that are quoted as normal are simply inadequate for optimal health. While most studies suggest that optimal levels should be maintained above 20–30 ng/dL, numerous studies show optimal benefit (reduced cancer and heart disease) at levels above 40-60 ng/dL. Adults should take 3-5000 IU a day. I have yet to see anyone taking 5000 IU a day reach unsafe levels. There is little chance of toxicity even though this recommendation is higher than you will see quoted by most experts. Take this amount for a few months, then get your level checked. Since Vitamin D enhances calcium absorption, I recommend you take vitamin K2 also, to help the calcium move into the bone and not accumulate in blood vessels.

Vitamin C

Most mammals make their own vitamin C. Humans, like a few other animals, do not synthesize their own vitamin C and it is thus an essential nutrient. Vitamin C is a very important antioxidant, helping us get rid of free-radicals, toxins, and to protect our cells from aging. Vitamin C also helps the absorption of iron and boosts the immune system. It is certainly possible to get plenty of vitamin C from the diet. Citrus, guava, kiwi, peppers, cantaloupe, papaya, and strawberries are all good sources of vitamin C, however a typical serving of these may only give you 50–100 mg of vitamin C. Some research would suggest that we need 10–20 times this amount (1000 – 2000 mg) a day. Spreading out your vitamin C intake throughout the day works best to provide your cells with this powerful antioxidant. Linus Pauling, winner of the Nobel prize in science, regularly took over 10,000 mg a day and lived into his 90's, though I do not recommend these mega-doses. Some recent work recommends a gram (1000 mg) daily along with ample fresh fruits and vegetables. When it comes to antioxidants, balance is important. We need an appropriate amount of them all (Vitamins E, C, A, and glutathione).

B-Vitamins

B-12 in particular, is vital for neurological function and, along with B6 and folate is vital for the methylation cycle that basically is responsible for building all protein, reading our DNA, and making neurotransmitters. Nothing could be more important, and if you are a vegetarian (a great way to eat a low toxin diet if it is organic) you will not get enough B-12 from your diet. If you are pregnant or nursing, the importance of supplementing B-12 for vegetarian moms cannot be overemphasized. I think it is wise to supplement vitamin B-12, folinic acid, vitamin B-6, and while you are at it, a little of all the B vitamins. This can be as a B-complex, or add B-12 with folate to your good multivitamin.

Multivitamin/Mineral Supplement

In my practice I offer a blood test called Spectracell micronutrient testing. This test involves spinning down tubes of blood and then analyzing the nutrient status of the WBCs (white blood cells). This gives us a window into the nutrients inside the cells. It is inside the cells that we need these nutrients to have proper health. There are good multivitamins that will probably cover your basic needs for most nutrients. In cases where you may be deficient, the amount of vitamins and nutrients in the multivitamin may not meet your specific needs. Nutrient deficiencies can be identified and treated. Testing and treating specific micronutrient deficiencies has been shown to reverse hypertension and heart disease. Many of us are deficient in certain minerals like calcium, magnesium, and zinc. It may be advisable to take a calcium/magnesium supplement with vitamin K2 to help with the movement of the calcium into the bone (your "bank account" for calcium).

Regardless of your diet and supplement regimen, micronutrient testing can provide a cell checkup and let you know which nutrients may not be effectively entering your cells. There are numerous factors that can interfere with nutrients entering the cell, such as absorption challenges, transport problems, health issues, and medications that alter nutrient movement and utilization. When we get the complete array of nutrients in the cells of our bodies, and add to that proper hormone levels, we start to experience optimal health and the vitality of youth.

Probiotics

Our intestinal tract is host to hundreds if not thousands of species of bacteria. These bacteria provide important functions for us, including breaking down foods further for better absorption, manufacturing certain vitamins, preventing disease, boosting the immune system and protecting us from toxicants. Fermented foods are a good source of natural probiotics (friendly bacteria). Most of us would benefit by taking a high-quality probiotic. This is one supplement where quality is especially important and not all probiotics are equal. In fact, I would advise against just buying the cheapest version of this supplement, as it either would have potentially no benefit or could even be harmful.

EXERCISE

You've probably heard "use it or lose it", right? Well this is true for our brains and true for our muscles. The use of our muscles provides many important values to us. If we build muscle, we increase our bone storage of calcium, which is important not only for the strength of the bones themselves, but for cell function throughout the body. There is greater improvement of bone density by sports and activities that involve the resistance to gravity. Swimming does provide benefit, but less so in the bone density area as it is relatively gravity neutral. Clearly, the heart health and lean mass benefits of swimming go far beyond what is measured in bone density.

By building our lean body mass (everything that is not fat), we increase our metabolic rate, and this helps us stay lean and feeling energetic. The hormone section of this book will be most pleasing to anyone who struggles with building muscle instead of fat. Having optimal thyroid and testosterone levels is miraculous for building muscle and losing fat, although it won't do you much good if all you do is sit or lie around. To build muscles, we must use them.

The good news is that no matter how sedentary you may have become, just starting to move will have huge dividends for you. You will notice the results in your energy and your strength within a month or two of starting your exercise.

What type of exercise should you do?

The best type of exercise is that which you will do! Seems logical but it's absolutely essential that you make a plan to start increasing, little by little, how much you exercise. I had let myself go so far that I had a BMI (body mass index) of 30 - the cutoff for obesity - and I was carrying over 60 lbs of fat. Don't get hung up on what your BMI is. Studies have shown that the waist-to-height ratio is even more important, so take a look in the mirror. If your waist (belly) is protruding, or if your dress size or belt size has been moving up, then it's time to make a change to reduce your health risks. Running was out of the question. So I started slowly walking a 2-mile loop near my house. Within a couple months I was able to add a few downhill slow jogs, and within a few more months, I was jogging the entire two miles (hills and all). I have recently been able to run the two miles at an 8 minute per mile pace. Less than a year before, I could barely walk this 2 mile course in 45 minutes.

If you have access to a pool and don't mind swimming or walking in the water, it can take some of the pressure off the joints. If you like to ride a bicycle, or play some sport, start slow and easy so you don't injure yourself, but get started. Perhaps you start with three times a week and then increase this when it doesn't hurt as much. When I started, it literally hurt to walk. Now that's ridiculous for an individual who was an athlete in high school. I had let myself go. Can anyone relate? The great news is that our body's cells are constantly turning over, so within a year you'll have all new cells anyway. This is true for many organs at least, like blood, skin, and intestinal lining.

Our brains are so precious, as they do not have the rapid turnover of cells that other parts of the body have. Ten percent of our fat cells turn over annually. A red blood cell's lifespan is 120 days, so you are constantly renewing your red blood cells. In fact, all cell lines from the bone marrow are in constant turnover. Since we cannot regenerate brain cells, I suggested at the beginning that we start off with taking care of any addictions. These are the most detrimental to our brains. Treat your brain like it is fragile. It is the precious powerhouse of your thoughts and emotions.

Testing For Toxins

There is now a good urine test that gives us a look inside your body at the levels of many key toxins. Other approaches look at hair excretion of toxins or actual levels of toxins in the blood. The hair analysis gives an idea of excretion over the time that hair has been growing. Knowing which toxins are being excreted at high levels will help you find ways to avoid the ongoing exposure to these toxins, and guides us in supporting their elimination. Remember, optimal health is all about getting the proper nutrients, avoiding toxins, and normalizing hormones that may be suppressed by toxins, age, stress, medications you may be taking, and past illness.

Summary of Health and Wellness

Address and conquer your addictions, always keeping this the number one priority if addictions have visited your life. If you use tobacco, get help and stop. If you use aspartame, stop immediately as this single move may add countless years to your life and save you from debilitating pain and suffering. Never drink or eat aspartame or substitute sweeteners. Change your eating habits to eat only organic, GMO-free whole foods, and avoid highly processed flour or sugar, as well as foods with artificial dyes and colors. Focus on vegetables, fruits, real meat, whole-grains, and whenever possible, free-range and organic foods. This will keep your insulin levels low and help you avoid the fat storage that happens with processed carbohydrates and insulin resistance.

Start exercising and continue to increase the amount and intensity, slowly at first to avoid injury.

Get your nutrients tested and take supplements to meet the needs. If testing is not available, take:

- 5000 IU a day vitamin D,
- 1000 mg a day Vitamin C (spread out during the day) if you can tolerate it. This may cause diarrhea.
- Vitamin B-12 with folinic acid or a B-complex
- Multivitamin
- Calcium/Magnesium with Vitamin K2
- Probiotic

Test your urine for toxins and work on eliminating as many sources of those toxins you seem to be having trouble with as possible.

You are now ready to add the hormone therapy.

Read on!

HORMONES

Hormones are chemical messengers created and released from endocrine glands into the blood to have an effect at a distant site through the activation of receptors. It is the specific receptors that determine which tissue or part of the body will respond to a given hormone. The term "hormone" was first used by Bayliss and Starling in 1902.

Hormones are able to coordinate physiology and metabolism regulating and controlling many different body functions. Hormones in many ways are much like neurotransmitters, the chemicals used by our nervous system and brain that allow us to think, and feel, form memories, and coordinate everything that our complex brain does.

Together with neurotransmitters, hormones essentially control all aspects of our body's physiology, biochemistry, and just about every aspect of our health and wellbeing. Just as the neurotransmitters serotonin, dopamine, and norepinephrine are critical in how our brain functions and how we feel, we have discovered that the thyroid hormones and sex hormones (testosterone, estrogen and progesterone) are critical in how we feel, having an equally profound effect on our mood.

Most people have heard of insulin resistance, where the receptors for insulin are not as responsive to the insulin in the blood stream. This triggers the body to make more insulin in an attempt to keep blood sugars normal, and in the process, we store more fat and gain weight.   A similar resistance at the receptors can occur for other hormones and explains why you can have hormone levels tested and be normal, yet you have the symptoms of that hormone being lacking.

So often the fatigue, anxiety or depression that you might have associated with aging or with addiction is no more than a hormonal deficiency. The good news is that once this is determined and your hormones are brought back to youthful levels, you can regain your energy and vitality.

Hormone replacement therapy for women who have either had surgical or age-related menopause has been a huge help in alleviating symptoms of sweats, fatigue, insomnia, poor energy, brain fog, and so much more. Sadly, the scare of the Women's Health Initiative (WHI) study, which showed increase in cardiovascular events for one arm of the study, has resulted in countless women dropping their hormone replacement therapy. Obesity may be a more significant risk factor and a variable not adequately considered in the WHI study. The reports of increased cardiovascular events were only in one arm of the study, where older women were taking synthetic progesterone. The entire study was with women on synthetic hormones.

Most women in menopause, and some before menopause, need not only estrogen and progesterone, but would benefit from optimal levels of DHEA and testosterone.

BIOLOGICALLY IDENTICAL HORMONES

If hormones are so vital to our health and the normal functioning of every cell in the body, would you want to replace these critical chemical messengers with synthetic, chemically-altered pharmaceutical molecules? Wouldn't you prefer chemical messengers that are identical to those that your body already makes?

You might wonder why a doctor would even prescribe a synthetic hormone if a natural, biologically identical option were available. The answer has to do with economics and politics. As a physician trained here in the USA at Dartmouth Medical School, I was adamant that I was trained by pure science and had the best education available in the world. I think that is still true, however, what I was not aware of for many years was the extent to which the pharmaceutical industry controls what research gets funded and published.

Biologically identical hormones are identical in structure to the natural hormones our bodies produce. Pharmaceutical companies cannot patent and make huge profits from molecules that are identical to our natural hormones. In order to make profits, the pharmaceutical companies intentionally synthesize molecules that are structurally different from our natural hormones. They can then patent these molecules and promote their use by doing research that shows benefits to health.

Since these synthetic, non-identical hormones will not have a perfect fit with the receptors, they often have serious side effects. We are all familiar with the numerous studies showing increased risk of breast cancer, heart attacks, strokes, pulmonary embolism, and Alzheimer's from the use of synthetic female hormones such as Premarin, Provera, and Prempro. Studies are showing comparatively improved safety when using bioidentical hormones. For hypothyroidism, the synthetic T4 thyroxin (levo-thyroxin) is the only option most physicians will give you. The natural biologically identical desiccated thyroid hormones that have been available for decades have fallen out of favor due to powerful marketing and lobbying from the pharmaceutical company manufacturing the T4 synthetic thyroid hormone. The use of just T4 has resulted in countless hypothyroid individuals being under treated and suffering the symptoms of hypothyroidism. New research is emerging supporting the use of combination T3/T4.

Where do the bio-identical natural hormones come from? They are extracted and synthesized from plants, typically soy and yams. With a prescription from an experienced physician, a compounding pharmacist can obtain pure biologically identical hormones and compound them into capsules, creams or other delivery methods. The use of pure pharmaceutical grade hormones micronized to provide maximum potency and good absorption results in hormone products that can restore you to youthful levels without the side effects typically seen with synthetic biologically altered pharmaceutical hormone products.

The medical literature supports the fact that many harmful effects are seen from the use of synthetic pharmaceutical products.

ADDICTION & HORMONES

Have you ever wondered if you drank too much, smoked too much, or should consider cutting back on your drinking, pot smoking, or use of pain medication/opiates or other drugs?

If you are pondering this question then the answer is a big YES!

This is a topic I know well as it has visited my family. If you regularly use opiates, alcohol, marijuana, or some other substance to help you get to sleep or to get through the day, then you likely are experiencing the effects this has on your hormones by the suppression of the pituitary, along with the energy–drain that results from addictions.

The first step to reclaiming your health and wellness is to tackle your addictions head on. Make this your number one priority. If you put conditions on this part of your journey, making excuses or reasons to delay dealing with your addiction, you likely will fail by falling right back into the addiction that has been sucking the very life out of you. This goes for cigarettes, alcohol, marijuana, pain pills, or opiates of any kind. Opiates for any reason are fine for short-term pain but a health disaster when used for over a month or two.

Take this part of your health journey as the KEY. It is a daily decision not to drink or use for that day. Take it one day at a time. Most of us cannot do this without professional help or without joining a 12–step program for the addiction we struggle with. You may need the help of an addiction physician or a drug and alcohol counselor. If you have been on opiates long term, you will need to taper off very slowly. This most often will require the guidance of an addiction specialist, and perhaps a prescription of Buprenorphine (Suboxone).

Think of your journey back to vibrant health like eating an artichoke. With each layer you take off, you get closer to the heart, where the real prize awaits you. We didn't get to this state of un-health overnight. Likewise, it will take some years to reclaim your health. Will it be worth it? ABSOLUTELY!

It turns out that there is good, solid, emerging evidence that drugs and alcohol suppress and shut down your master hormone gland, the pituitary. The pituitary sends key messages to your thyroid, adrenal glands, testes (men), ovaries (women), bones, muscles, and pancreas. With all these major endocrine organs shutting down, it's no wonder you feel tired, listless, depressed, anxious, weak, sleep deprived, and disinterested in sex. It is no surprise that you have basically lost that spark of life you once had as a child.

I stumbled on this information working in my addiction clinic. One of my 25 year old patients asked if I would check his testosterone. "Doc, just humor me and check my testosterone. I was reading online that the symptoms of testosterone deficiency match mine exactly". You see, this young man was so ravaged by anxiety and depression that his psychiatrist had tried multiple SSRI antidepressants, Cymbalta, Wellbutrin, amitriptyline, seroquel, and many others with little benefit. He had tried group treatment, individual therapy. He had been unable to work, leave the house or go into a store for almost a year and was hospitalized once for extreme suicidal thoughts, which had been with him the entire year.

Imagine my surprise to find his total testosterone level below 200 (optimal for his age is 600-1200) and his free testosterone below 50 (optimal for his age is 150-240). With correction of his testosterone levels, he was back to work in a month and feeling 90% better within a few months. I started checking hormone levels on all of my addiction and opiate-dependent patients who were symptomatic, and most had very low testosterone.

It appears that toxins in our environment and drugs and alcohol suppress the anterior pituitary, our master hormone gland. It's no wonder, why persons addicted to drugs and alcohol have such a hard time quitting. You see; the fatigue and low energy that accompanies both withdrawal and low hormone levels is briefly and temporarily made better by using the drugs or alcohol, only to further deplete neurotransmitters and suppress hormone production.

We don't know yet how long it will take for a pituitary suppressed by drugs and/or alcohol to return to normal. One thing for certain is that it will return to normal function in most cases, if allowed to heal. In order to heal, the recovering persons can have their hormones supported naturally with biologically identical hormones, allowing them to wean off or stop taking the substance (drug or alcohol) that is gradually killing them.

Attempting to stop drinking or using drugs, will require more than willpower for most people. I encourage addiction prevention counseling and 12–step programs which are available in most cities of the world and are anonymous and free of charge. In many cases, such as an opiate addiction or dependence, there are tools such as the medication Suboxone (Buprenorphine) that can be given as a slow taper to assist in the process of getting off opiates completely.

For many opiate users, I hear the story over and over: "Doc, you don't understand, I have real pain". My experience has been that that nearly 100% of these "pain patients" get better (have less pain) as we wean off the opiates. You see, opiates are wonderful for short-term pain, and a very poor option for chronic pain. Tolerance develops, just as it does for the heroin addict or pain pill addict, causing the need for increasing doses of the opiate to get the same effect. The brain creates new opiate receptors in the face of all these opiates, and opiate receptors are pain receptors. Now you experience severe pain when the pain stimulus is minimal.

Eventually, the opiates stop working. At this point most addicts will take the opiates just to not get sick and go through the horrible opiate withdrawal symptoms. Opiate withdrawal mimics the worst flu, with sweats, shakes, twitches, goose bumps, rapid heart rate, high blood pressure, restlessness, body aches, and unbearable anxiety. While the acute withdrawal symptoms subside in a few days or so, most are left lethargic, depressed, and anxious, with cravings that last for months and months.

Correcting the suppressed hormones with natural biological identical hormones allows you to feel much less anxious, improves energy and mood, and removes many of the symptoms that we once attributed to withdrawal.

Now you can become drug free and then, for most, wean off the hormone replacements as your pituitary returns to normal function.

HEALTHY AGING & HORMONES

There is a steady decline in all of our hormone levels as we age. In women, the decline of estrogen and progesterone is commonly referred to as menopause. What is now understood is that men also suffer from a decline in hormones, called andropause by some. Some physicians think of this as natural, the expected decline associated with aging. The truth of the matter is that we can replace hormones naturally and return older individuals to the vitality and cellular health of a much younger age. Due to the extreme pressures on our endocrine system from environmental toxins, we are now seeing hormone suppression never before experienced by humans. The improved quality of life is one most will embrace and wonder how they ever managed before.

"Normal" when it comes to hormone levels, is a lab designation of what is usual for age. In other words, a male 60 years old could have a testosterone level less than 20% that of a 20 year old but have that fall in the "normal" range. For a woman after menopause, estrogen and progesterone levels can fall near zero and be considered "normal." A key principle in real preventative medicine is the concept of using biological identical hormones to bring levels near those for a young adult.

Along with hormone levels falling as we age comes a resistance to hormones at the receptor such that normal hormone levels can have little effect on the target tissues. In some cases there is also a relative lack or abundance of a transport protein, such as sex steroid binding globulins, meaning that relatively little of a hormone like testosterone is able to reach the receptors. In the case of thyroid hormone, there can be a relative abundance of thyroid binding globulin such that there is inadequate free-T3 and free-T4 to have normal thyroid function. The interplay between hypothalamic, pituitary and thyroid T3 production is complex.

When it comes to hormone replacement, it is best to treat the patient and not just the hormone levels. It is possible to have normal levels of thyroid hormone, but feel all the symptoms of fatigue, weight gain, brittle nails, dry skin, hair loss, etc. We use lab values to get us in the range, and use symptoms to fine-tune our hormone replacement.

Estrogen, progesterone and thyroid hormones have been replaced for decades, but there is now a growing understanding of the synergistic benefit of optimizing all hormones. Indeed, the typical diseases associated with aging, like diabetes, heart disease, hypertension and cancers, can be reduced by restoring a healthy immune system and hormone balance.

To be certain your hormone replacement does not put you at increased risk of adverse events and side effects, you should only use biologically identical hormones. In order to know your natural hormones are effective, it is wise to have your levels monitored, and the improvement in energy, mood, and symptoms should confirm for you that you are on the right path.

HYPOTHALAMIC-PITUITARY HORMONES

The Master Hormone Gland

The Pituitary is a tiny 1 cm gland sitting at the base of the brain in the tiny pituitary fossa called the sella turcica, just above the sphenoid sinus. While the pituitary can be considered the master gland, it is also under very tight control from releasing hormones (factors) by the hypothalamus and is subject to negative feedback by the circulating hormones in the body.

For simplicity and clarity, the following diagram shows the hypothalamus/pituitary (in the brain) releasing TSH to the thyroid, ACTH to the adrenals, FSH to testes and ovaries, and LH to ovaries.

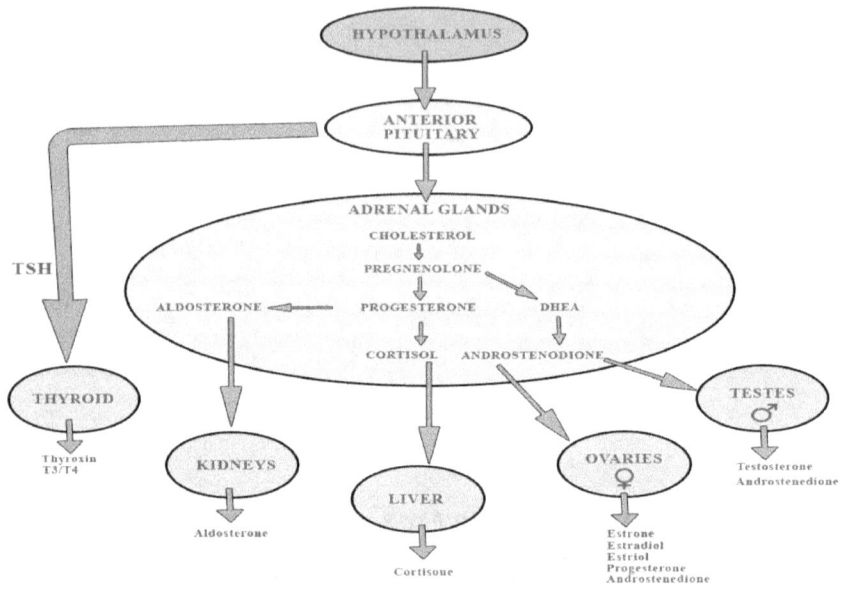

TSH - stimulates the Thyroid gland -releases thyroid hormones T3/T4

ACTH - stimulates the Adrenal gland -releases cortisol

FSH / LH to Testes - releases Testosterone

FSH / LH to Ovaries - releases Estrogen & Progesterone

Circulating thyroid hormone will signal the pituitary to release less TSH.

Circulating cortisol will signal the pituitary to release less ACTH.

Circulating testosterone will signal the pituitary to releases less FSH and LH.

Circulating estrogen and progesterone will signal less FSH and LH.

While the exact mechanisms by which the function of the pituitary is shut down by aging, addictions, and toxins is not well known, the effects of this are easily seen in blood tests for these hormones. When it's the pituitary that is affected and the hormones of the pituitary are low, you see low levels of TSH, FSH, and LH. When pituitary hormones are low and there is a resultant decrease in hormones from their target organs (thyroid, adrenal, testes and ovaries), a subsequent decrease in the negative feedback to the hypothalamus-pituitary occurs. This is how the body keeps a balance and tries to increase production of these vital hormones. It thus takes a skilled assessment of symptoms along with hormone values to get a clear picture.

THYROID HORMONE

Since the addition of iodine to salt in the 1920's in the USA, this major cause of hypothyroidism (low thyroid function) has been removed. Despite this, for various reasons low thyroid function may be affecting 30 to 40% of the population. Well over 100 symptoms are attributed to low functioning thyroid.

Thyrotropin Releasing Hormone (TRH) from the hypothalamus triggers the release of Thyrotropin (Thyroid Stimulating Hormone-TSH) from the anterior pituitary. TSH then stimulates the thyroid to produce thyroid hormone. The thyroid initially produces T4, which is much more abundant than the biologically active T3. If all is working perfectly, then up to 80% of T4 is converted to T3. Most of the T4 and T3 are carried in the blood, bound to proteins. The biologically active forms of thyroid hormone are the free-T3 and free-T4, which represents 0.3% and 0.02% respectively of the total thyroid hormone in the blood.

The recent reliance on the tests TSH and T4 by physicians without paying attention to the symptoms of the patient in front of them or the free-T3 test, leaves this condition sadly under appreciated, causing much needless suffering. Many patients who are being treated for low thyroid are only given synthetic T4 (synthroid, L-thyroxine). This will suppress the TSH, making it look like the patient has normal thyroid function, but if there is inadequate free-T3, you can have normal labs and continue to suffer from hypothyroidism.

Free-T3 (and to a lesser extent free-T4) is vital for the energy (think heat) production of every cell in the body, increasing mitochondrial oxidative metabolism driven by ATP utilization via ATPase activity. With reduced ATP, every cell in the body may be functioning at less than optimal capacity. It is this universal need for thyroid hormone that makes free-T3 necessary for almost any body organ or system.

If the cells in the brain are slowed, you may experience mental confusion, slow speech, forgetfulness, depression, anxiety, nervousness, emotional instability, sleeplessness, poor concentration, poor memory, and fatigue. One has to wonder if there may be a connection with all the increased ADD, ADHD, autism, etc. that we see these days. Heavy metal and toxins may also interfere with formation of T3.

At the level of muscles and joints, we see weakness, fatigue, lethargy, lack of energy, joint and muscle pains or swelling, and arthritis. Chronic fatigue syndrome (CFS) and fibromyalgia have been improved with natural thyroid hormone replacement.

If the cells of the immune system are affected, you see increased allergies and increased infections such as colds, sinus infections, lung infections, and more. A strong association in the early 1900's was seen with tuberculosis (TB) infections and hypothyroidism.

When cells of the integument (skin, intestinal lining) are involved, you see cold hands and feet, hair loss, thinning of the eyebrows or eyelashes, dry skin, tingling or itchy skin, decreased sweating, pallor or puffy skin, brittle fingernails with ridging, and constipation (slower, infrequent bowel movements). In severe deficiencies of thyroid hormone (adult myxedema or childhood cretinism) the tongue can be thickened, the hands pudgy, and the skin eczema-like being dry, and coarse.

The thyroid hormones seem to interact with the other steroid (sex) hormones such that being low thyroid for a woman can contribute to miscarriages and infertility. For both men and women, low thyroid can cause reduced libido.

Fatigue and difficulty losing weight seem to be the most common symptoms for adults with low thyroid. Since every cell in the body is affected by a lowered energy and metabolic rate, it is no wonder that weight gain is common, and fatigue is such a prominent part. Imagine every cell of your body running at 60-70% or worse!

Prior to the 1970's when blood tests for thyroid hormone were developed, doctors would have you take your basal temperature (oral or under arm) when you first wake up, before you even get out of bed. A normal temperature is 97.8 to 98.2 and a temperature over 98.2 might indicate you are ill, or, if you are on thyroid hormones, could represent too high of a dose or that you are hyperthyroid.

In hormone therapy, it is best to use TSH levels and free-T3, along with how the patient is feeling. If the symptoms are resolving, you may be at the right dose. If the TSH is below 0.1-0.3, the dose is too high and it is advisable to use just enough to get normal function, but still retain some natural thyroid function.

Hypothyroidism has been associated with migraines and other headaches, emotional and behavioral issues, hypertension, heart attacks and atherosclerosis, and many of the complications associated with diabetes, which are thought to be due to atherosclerosis and blood vessel damage.

Make sure your doctor checks your free-T3 along with the TSH. Focus on symptoms and not just lab values. Many of us have normal or even high levels of circulating thyroid hormones, but due to receptor resistance, we have the symptoms of low thyroid function.

SYMPTOMS OF TOO MUCH THYROID MEDICINE (HYPERTHYROID)

- Nervousness, tremor
- Sweating, hot
- Heart palpitations, rapid heart rate

SYMPTOMS OF LOW THYROID

- Fatigue, tired
- Weak, low energy and motivation
- Depression, anxiety, irritability
- Cold
- Weight gain, increased body fat
- Poor memory and mood, brain fog
- Cognitive impairment, poor concentration
- Thin sparse hair, thin skin and nails, eyebrows
- High cholesterol, heart disease
- Frequent infections (colds, sinus, ears, throat, lungs)
- Constipation
- Fluid retention
- Arthritis, fibromyalgia, chronic fatigue syndrome
- Numbness and tingling, itchy skin especially hands and feet and in winter
- Menstrual issues, miscarriages

BENEFITS OF NORMALIZING THYROID

- Improved energy and strength
- Improved mood and sense of well-being
- Improved memory and cognition
- Menstrual regularity
- Improved hair, nails and skin
- Less fat and normal body temperature
- Less depression and anxiety
- Less atherosclerosis and heart disease
- Regular bowel movements

DHEA / STEROID HORMONES

DHEA (dehydroepiandrosterone) is a steroid hormone derived from cholesterol.

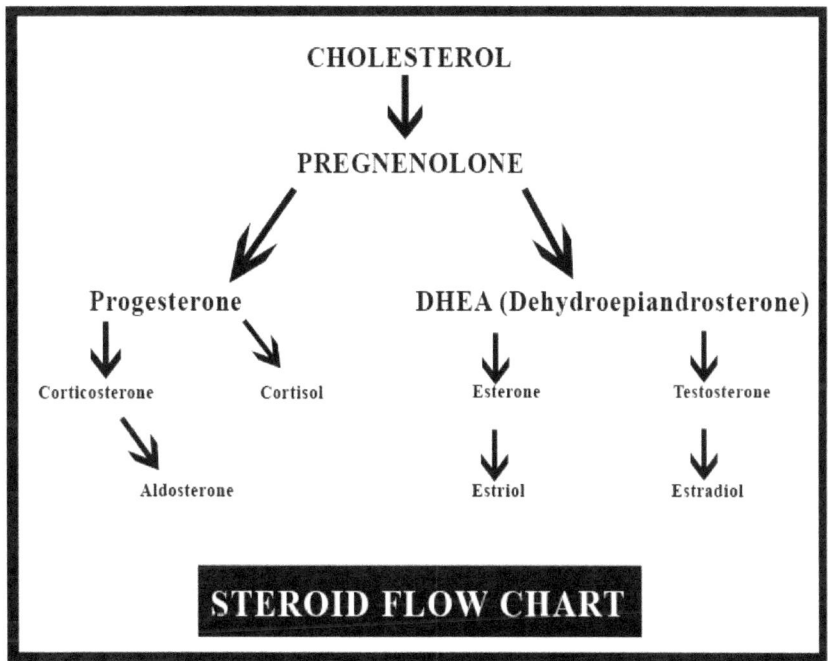

DHEA is a precursor of testosterone and estrogen. While it was once thought to have limited value by itself, studies have now shown that it decreases with age, and low DHEA is associated with higher rates of cancer and heart disease. It seems having optimal levels of DHEA helps the immune system, brain function, and energy levels, and seems to reduce insulin sensitivity. By reducing insulin sensitivity,

DHEA helps with weight control and protects the body from the damaging effects of high insulin states. DHEA has antioxidant properties and helps with cellular metabolism.

Because of the conversion of DHEA to testosterone and estrogen, its use must be carefully monitored. It is especially important to use extreme caution in women and children, and not to use DHEA if you might be pregnant.

When supplementing DHEA, it is best to take a micronized, sustained release, compounded pharmaceutical preparation. Over the counter supplements may contain impurities, have unknown potency, and have a short half-life that would require dosing three to four times a day.

BENEFITS OF DHEA

- Decreases visceral fat
- Decreases cholesterol
- Improved immune system
- Lowers cardiovascular risk
- Improves memory and mood
- Improves energy
- Restores sexual vitality
- Prevents osteoporosis (increases bone density)
- Reduces lipid peroxidation (acts like antioxidant) reduces insulin requirement
- Enhances the immune system (T-cell activation)
- Reduces inflammation
- An important precursor for many hormones

TESTOSTERONE IN MEN

Just as women go through menopause, it is now understood that the typical man has such a profound loss of testosterone function with age that this can be considered andropause. Men make testosterone in the testes in response to FSH from the pituitary. The pituitary can be suppressed by natural aging, by drug or alcohol abuse, by environmental toxins, or by disease. The typical testosterone levels for a man in his 70's or 80's are so low that most would not be able to maintain an erection. By age 50, all men are typically experiencing the loss of muscle strength and tone, not to mention fatigue, depression, anxiety and mental decline, and loss of libido. We now know that this is in part due to low testosterone levels.

Testosterone has now been shown to benefit the heart and reduce cardiovascular risk factors. It reduces inflammation with lower CRP and higher HDL (the good cholesterol). Past studies that showed a negative effect of testosterone on lipids were based on synthetic and oral testosterone that interfered with the liver. Natural testosterone replacement with bio-identical testosterone does not harm and actually has tremendous benefits to longevity and heart health. It is now believed that men with testosterone levels below 300 ng/dL deserve to have testosterone replacement therapy.

Testosterone reduces obesity, raises lean muscle mass, lowers bad cholesterol, and raises the good cholesterol, thus reducing heart disease and strokes. Studies have also shown a decrease in the cognitive decline of Alzheimer's disease, and improved lifespan.

There has been much controversy in the literature about the possible link of testosterone with prostate cancer and other cancers. Studies looking at natural testosterone replacement have consistently shown testosterone to be protective against cancers. That being said, because it is an anabolic steroid (stimulates growth), it is advisable to check a PSA before starting testosterone replacement, and not to start taking testosterone if you have a high PSA, or have any other active cancer. A high PSA may indicate that you have prostate cancer.

Natural bio-identical testosterone is available in a pharmaceutical injection, and in gels, creams, patches, and underarm applications. It can also be compounded for topical application. Testosterone is a controlled substance.

Extreme caution is needed if the person using testosterone as a cream, gel, or topical application is to come in contact with women or children. It is particularly important to completely avoid accidental transfer of your testosterone to a pregnant woman. If your partner might be pregnant or may become pregnant, I recommend either the shots (that cannot be transferred by contact), or apply the cream in the morning and take a shower after work and before you might be amorous with your lady. The patch also provides protection against accidental transfer.

SYMPTOMS OF LOW TESTOSTERONE IN MEN

- Fatigue
- Depression
- Anxiety / irritability
- Low sense of well-being
- Lack of assertiveness / drive
- Weakness (decreased muscle strength)
- Less endurance
- Poor libido (ultimately inability to get or maintain erections)
- Increased fat
- Sleep issues
- Increased infections (poor immune system)
- Poor memory
- Tendon and joint problems
- Thin skin

BENEFITS OF TESTOSTERONE IN MEN

- Less fatigue, depression, anxiety (greater well-being)
- Increased muscle strength and endurance
- Decreased body fat
- Improved memory
- Decreased cholesterol and heart disease
- Improves skin and connective tissue (faster healing)
- Improved libido and sexual performance
- Protects cardiovascular, musculoskeletal and immune systems
- Increased RBCs from bone marrow (better oxygen carrying capacity)
- Increased metabolism by increased conversion of thyroid T4 to active T3
- Protects against diabetes, MS, and cancers (don't take when you have active cancer)

TESTOSTERONE IN WOMEN

Once a woman is past the age of child bearing, and especially after menopause, there is a significant decline in testosterone, just as there is for men. Women make testosterone in the adrenals and ovaries, and typically have levels about 1/10th those of men. If you have had a hysterectomy/oophorectomy and no longer have ovaries, then your production of testosterone is even lower.

Testosterone for women has the same important role of increased strength and bone density, increased libido, and less fatigue, depression and, anxiety.

For many women (and most after menopause) the combination of low estrogen, low progesterone, and low testosterone is especially difficult. The presence of sex binding globulin that binds most if not all the free testosterone makes the little that remains unavailable to the receptors. It is no wonder that most have lost interest in sex and are just tired, depressed, anxious, and unmotivated. Interests drift to more sedentary activities.

Testosterone supplementation for post-menopausal women can be done carefully with very low-dose compounded creams. Levels should be carefully monitored, as the side effects of testosterone levels that are too high in women can be permanent, such as the lowering of the voice, or hair growth in unwanted places.

Women who were testosterone deficient will experience numerous benefits from testosterone replacement, including improved strength, bone density, energy, mood, and libido, along with improved skin tone and protection against cardiovascular disease and Alzheimer's disease. They will also benefit from lower cholesterol and higher HDL (the good cholesterol).

Just as with men, when supplementing with topical bio-identical natural testosterone creams or gels, it is important that this is not accidentally transferred to younger women who could be pregnant or to children.

You should check levels of free testosterone and total testosterone monthly until you are certain the dose is correct.

SYMPTOMS OF LOW TESTOSTERONE IN WOMEN

- Fatigue
- Low energy
- Increased body fat
- Decreased muscle mass
- Decreased metabolism
- Poor endurance
- Low sex drive & libido
- Thin skin with less collagen
- Wrinkles

BENEFITS OF TESTOSTERONE IN WOMEN
(Do not give if pregnant or can become pregnant.)

- Improved energy and well being
- Improved strength and endurance
- More muscle and less fat
- Less heart disease and diabetes
- Improved sexual function
- Improved skin texture and thickness
- Less wrinkles

ESTROGEN/PROGESTERONE

To make sense of estrogen and progesterone levels, it's important to understand the variation in female hormones that occurs in the monthly cycle prior to menopause. Below, you see the spikes mid-cycle of LH (luteinizing hormone) and FSH (follicle stimulating hormone) that are secreted from the anterior pituitary and trigger ovulation in women prior to menopause. Mid-cycle, corresponding to the spikes in LH and FSH, there is a rise in estradiol (estrogen) and progesterone spikes during the last half of the month as the uterine lining prepares for possible implantation should a fertilized ovum attach.

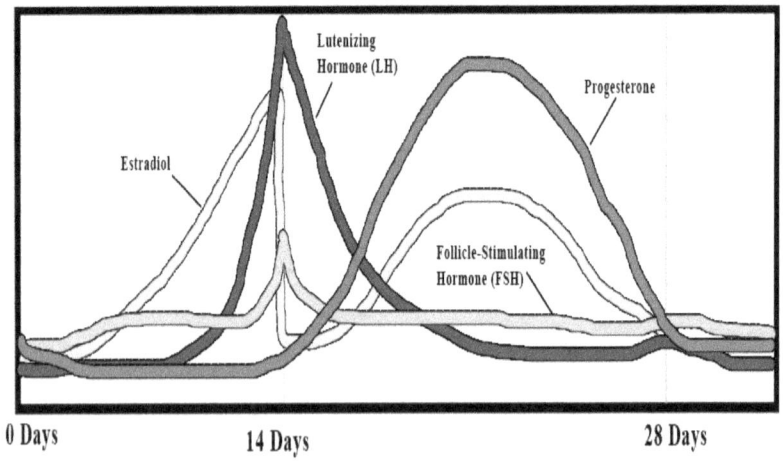

The typical menstrual cycle lasts 28 days, with day one being the start of menstruation. Estradiol continues to rise for the first 14 days stimulating growth and thickening of the uterine lining to prepare for possible pregnancy. In the middle of the month one ovary will release an egg (ovulation) and the remaining follicle starts producing progesterone and a little testosterone. The last two weeks the uterus prepares for pregnancy, the primary role of progesterone, which remains high for the last two weeks of the cycle. Progesterone's name literally means "promoting gestation," meaning pregnancy. If the egg was not fertilized, no pregnancy occurs and at the end of the month the uterine lining sloughs off in what is known as your period.

In the years before menopause, you can see that hormone levels vary greatly depending on the time in a woman's menstrual cycle. There is a gradual decline of progesterone starting in the mid thirties, and after menopause estrogen levels fall precipitously.

During pregnancy, the uterus produces progesterone and levels are as much as 20 times pre-pregnancy levels. Have you ever wondered why you felt so good during pregnancy? Have you ever heard of postpartum depression? After a baby is born there is an immediate and dramatic fall in progesterone levels. This results in a relatively high amount of estrogen when compared to progesterone. When estrogen levels are high (as in pregnancy, especially postpartum, birth control pills, artificial estrogens being taken), the liver produces increased thyroid binding globulin (TBG). While you may have normal levels of thyroid hormones, you may be experiencing the symptoms of low thyroid as the active free thyroid (free-T3 and free-T4) are inadequate. Low thyroid hormone function (functional hypothyroidism) can occur even when levels are "normal".

The section on thyroid has addressed the importance of treating the patient (symptoms), and not the labs.

It's the balance of estrogen and progesterone that is key here. Progesterone increases metabolism and thus promotes weight loss, mobilizes fluid, decreases swelling, thins the blood (thus preventing blood clots), stimulates new bone formation, and enhances the function of the thyroid hormones. Estrogen promotes fat storage and weight gain, fluid retention, thickening of the blood (increasing the risk of blood clots), reduces the availability of the thyroid hormones, and slows bone loss.

It is estrogen dominance that is the main issue creating a list of symptoms bringing women to the doctors.

ESTROGEN DOMINANCE SYMPTOMS

- Severe menstrual cramps and heavy periods
- Endometriosis, ovarian cysts, uterine fibroids
- Irregular menstrual cycles
- Infertility and multiple   miscarriages
- Premenstrual headaches, mood swings, breast tenderness, fluid retention
- Anxiety, panic attacks, depression
- Migraines
- Low energy and low sex drive

Some of these symptoms overlap with the effects of physiologic hypothyroidism discussed earlier, and some may be affected by relative low testosterone as well.

Women suffering from the symptoms of estrogen dominance are often offered a hysterectomy (with or without the removal of the ovaries – to prevent future ovarian cancer) or synthetic hormone therapy. While natural hormone therapy will not protect you from becoming pregnant, it can help with most of the above issues and greatly enhance your mood, energy, and wellbeing.

Estrogen levels fall off precipitously at menopause and the classic symptoms begin: hot flashes, insomnia, anxiety, depression, poor concentration, vaginal dryness, loss of libido, weakness, dry thin hair, wrinkled sagging skin, and an increase risk for heart disease, stroke, bone loss, and Alzheimer's. If you are a woman without estrogen, either from menopause or surgical menopause from a hysterectomy, you should take estrogen. It is ideal to take natural estrogen (not synthetic), and to optimize levels to those of a younger woman.

Progesterone levels also fall off as a woman ages. They lose the critical balance needed between estrogen and progesterone, especially if they are getting an estrogen prescription but no progesterone. Most doctors prescribe synthetic medroxy-progesterone (Provera) and this is a completely different molecule that has been shown in numerous studies to have serious side effects, including birth defects (should not be given in pregnancy), increased risk of breast cancer, increased risk of heart disease, and elevated cholesterol. Natural progesterone provides a long list of benefits without any of these negative side effects.

Progesterone helps balance estrogen dominance and alleviates PMS symptoms; irritability, headaches, and mood swings. Progesterone also helps with the typical menopausal symptoms while protecting against heart disease, cancer, osteoporosis, and protect against the symptoms of estrogen excess listed above.

For women on hormone replacement, there is the issue of whether or not to have a menstrual cycle. If you stop your progesterone for a week, you mimic the natural cycle and that drop of progesterone will trigger bleeding. If you wish to get pregnant, this is an important renewal process for the uterus. Studies seem to suggest, that it is not necessary to menstruate regularly, especially for women of menopausal age.

BENEFITS OF ESTROGEN IN WOMEN

- Less fatigue
- Less depression
- Improved mood
- Improved libido
- Protects against urogenital atrophy
- Less skin atrophy and wrinkles
- Less heart disease
- Fewer strokes
- Less colon cancer
- Less osteoporosis
- Fewer UTIs
- Less Alzheimer's disease
- Less macular degeneration
- Protects against cataracts

BENEFITS OF PROGESTERONE IN WOMEN
(Do not take if pregnant or can become pregnant.)

- Reduces PMS symptoms
- Improved mood
- Improved urogenital integrity
- Less heart disease
- Protects against breast cancer
- Less osteoporosis
- Moderates effects of excess estrogen
- Less fluid retention and Less bloating
- Less headaches
- Less bleeding (menstrual cycle related)
- Fewer fibroids

MELATONIN

Melatonin is a hormone secreted by the tiny pineal gland in the brain. It is formed from serotonin, with increased production when the sun goes down (the lights are off), showing a circadian rhythm.

The pineal gland has recently been shown to be a master gland in mediating and promoting the immune system, and melatonin is also now known to be an important and powerful antioxidant.

Melatonin is known to help promote sleep, along with its immune benefits and ability to help the body rid itself of toxins. This is a supplement that we probably all should consider taking. Numerous studies have now shown its ability to protect the body from the toxic effects of heavy metals like the aluminum that is found in so many vaccines, drugs of abuse (like meth-amphetamine), and other known toxins.

Young children should not take more than 1 mg, and adults appear to be able to safely take up to 10 mg or more though there is some controversy about this.
If the dose is too high and you are using a slow release (long acting version), then you may awaken in the morning a little sleepy. You can take a lower dose or take your dose earlier in the evening if this happens.

Melatonin has been known to stimulate the melanocytes (the cells that make pigment) in some animals. It can lighten the color of frogs, and some elderly people have noticed some return of blond hair where hair had been white.

In this toxic world we live in, the main role for melatonin is that of helping detoxify and boosting the immune system, making us less vulnerable to infections and cancers. Melatonin also reduces the metabolic syndrome by reducing insulin resistance and fat storage.

VITAMIN D3

Vitamin D3, cholecalciferol, is actually a sterol hormone, and is the only "vitamin" that cannot be obtained just from the diet.

Vitamin D's classic role is for bone and calcium metabolism. Severe Vitamin D deficiency, in children, causes rickets, with poor mineralization of the bones, bowing of the legs, and prominence around the costochondral junctions of the chest. In adults, severe deficiency causes demineralization of the bones, increased fractures, low calcium, and increased alkaline phosphatase activity.

Hundreds of studies are now pointing to other important roles for vitamin D. It is believed that it assists in protecting against heart disease, dementia, cancer, mood and depression issues, along with immune system benefits and the known protective benefits for bones. There are ongoing studies looking at its possible role in the protection of normal brain development and possible protection against autism.

This is one supplement you should absolutely be taking and in amounts much greater than previously thought. The Academy of Pediatrics just increased the recommendation to 800–1200 IU a day, but I find this level of supplementation to be borderline for most infants and toddlers and totally inadequate for school age to adults. I took 5000 IU daily faithfully for a couple years and my level was 49. After a couple more years of perhaps taking the 5000 IU twice a week, my level had dropped to 17! I suspect 5000 IU daily will be appropriate for most teens and adults.

I would not recommend over 10,000 IU a day for more than a few months without checking your level. Vitamin D is a fat-soluble vitamin and as such it potentially could accumulate to toxic levels, where there may be a tendency to develop high calcium and kidney stones.

Along with fish oil (one teaspoon or five gel caps daily) and a good multivitamin/mineral supplement with antioxidants and B-vitamins, vitamin D3 should be the cornerstone of everyone's health program when it comes to supplementing vital nutrients.

GROWTH HORMONE

I do not use growth hormone in my practice. This hormone, while having many potential benefits, is very tightly regulated due to its powerful effects and its abuse by body builders and some athletes. In a way it is unfortunate that small physiologic doses are not made more available as many people undoubtedly suffer from deficiency of this hormone. Access to growth hormone is only available through an endocrinologist, who can do specific tests to determine if you are severely deficient in growth hormone.

SYMPTOMS OF HORMONE DEFICIENCY
LOW HUMAN GROWTH HORMONE (HGH)

- Low energy
- Fatigue
- Poor concentration
- Memory challenges
- Depression
- Anxiety / irritability
- Poor sleep
- Lack of ambition / initiative / drive
- Decreased sense of well-being
- Low blood sugar
- Low blood pressure (BP can be high in extreme stress)
- Poor immunity / increased infections
- Poor muscle development
- Decreased endurance
- Excess abdominal body fat
- Poor healing
- Osteoporosis (decreased bone mass)
- Increased wrinkles and thin hair and nails
- Increased insulin resistance / hyperlipidemia
- Atherosclerosis (cardiovascular disease)
- Infertility
- Headaches
- Low libido
- Irregular menstrual cycles

BENEFITS OF GROWTH HORMONE REPLACEMENT
(Not currently available in most States)

- Improved cardiovascular function
- Decreased atherosclerosis
- Increased energy and exercise capacity
- Increased muscle size and strength
- Improved stamina
- Improved libido
- Less anxiety
- Less depression
- Decreased fat
- Increased bone mass and growth
- Improved hair and nails
- Improved memory
- Less anxiety
- Less depression
- Improved happiness / mood
- Improved wound healing and protein synthesis
- Increased REM stage IV sleep
- Improved sense of well-being
- Increased immunity (less cancer / less infections)
- Improved skin (less wrinkles)

THE GOALS / LAB VALUES

It is important that you realize most doctors would not consider optimal levels of hormones or nutrients to be necessary nor even advisable. To optimize hormone function, one aims for the high end of normal for ages 20-30. Since these values vary from lab to lab, this area requires that you see a physician who understands how to interpret the lab values that you get. Since normal ranges are established based on the local population serviced by a lab, and our population as a whole, is deficient in many hormones, you can start to appreciate the difficulty in interpreting the "normal" ranges that the labs provide to doctors.

These results can vary based on the time of day you draw them, and the timing in relation to when you may have taken certain hormone supplements. The PSA can be artificially raised by recent sexual activity or bike riding that can massage the prostate. For women, the use of birth control pills or natural hormone replacements will have major effects on the levels of the steroid (sex) hormones (estrogen, progesterone) and the FSH and LH from the pituitary.

Following, I list one suggestion for which labs to get done as you begin to look at the hormone function. Some practitioners are using saliva tests. The labs below are for blood levels of these hormones, which I find to be less variable and thus more reliable.

RECOMMENDED LAB DRAWS:

Men–Initial:
      DHEA, free and total testosterone, free T3, free-T4, TSH, FSH, LH, Vit D3, lipid panel, CMP, CBC, PSA, prolactin.

Men-Follow-up:
      Free and total testosterone, free-T3, TSH, DHEA (others as indicated clinically)

Women-Initial:
      DHEA, free and total testosterone, free-T3, free-T4, TSH, FSH, LH, Vit D3, lipid panel, CBC, CMP, prolactin, progesterone, estradiol.

Women Follow-up:
      DHEA, Free and total Testosterone, free-T3, TSH, estradiol, progesterone (others as indicated clinically)

SUMMARY

Despite the tremendous advances in medicine of the past century, the importance of maintaining optimal hormone levels based on function, and not just on lab results, may be a lost art for most physicians today. We live in a much more toxic environment than ever before. Endocrine disruptors are all around us. Such toxins can be passed on from one generation to the next through altered genetic material. The Endocrinology Society of America has recently written about toxicant induced loss of tolerance (TILT) and is becoming aware of the greater extent to which toxins may alter hormone function. TILT is a theory where toxicants make a person sensitive to previously tolerated chemicals, drugs, foods or hormones. This means we can no longer rely on lab values, but must take a careful history and examine the patient, much like doctors once did decades ago when lab results were not available.

We now recognize insulin resistance, where insulin levels can be normal (and often high) and yet there is resistance to the normal function of that insulin at the receptor on the cells. We must be alert to similar patterns of normal or even high hormone levels, where the hormones are not functioning well at the cellular level. Thyroid is an important example, as it now appears that a growing percentage of the population may be suffering from thyroid deficiency despite normal lab values. In the case of the thyroid, it is also important that we check the free-T3 and TSH, but not assume that the thyroid function is normal just because the labs may be normal.

While hormone replacement therapy is desperately needed to improve longevity and quality of life for the elderly, I also believe a significant portion of children and younger adults suffer from poor functioning hormones or frank hormone deficiencies.

Our goal should be optimal health and wellbeing for all. I wish this for the unborn child growing in her mother's womb, for every newborn and child, and every living person. To safely navigate the toxic world we now find ourselves in, I firmly believe there are a few key factors:

1. Avoid toxins: this includes eating GMO-free and organic. This also includes avoiding certain vaccines like the current Dtap if pregnant, which contains 330 micrograms of aluminum.
2. Supplement deficiencies: at least Vitamin D3, and for pregnancy, a prenatal and fish oil, and for vegetarians, B12, and most of us will benefit from added nutrients.
3. Get regular exercise.
4. Build a loving community for your family, minimizing stress.
5. Replace hormone deficiencies with natural bio-identical hormones.
6. Live in gratitude, free of resentments and full of wonder.

WISHING YOU HEALTH, PEACE, LOVE, AND
HAPPINESS,

Dr. Paul

Contact: **www.Naturaintegrativemedicine.com**

For your personal Hormone & Nutrient Optimization
approach to restoring health.

REFERENCES

Introduction

1. http://www.integrativepediatricsonline.com/blog/
2. http://www.thelancet.com/journals/lancet/article/PIIS01 40-6736(13)61611-6/abstract
3. http://www.integrativepediatricsonline.com/blog/2013/0 8/19/b-12-and-homocysteine-the-key-to-heart-disease-stroke-and-other-blood-clots/
4. http://healingfromdepression.com
5. http://www.integrativepediatricsonline.com/blog/2013/0 4/29/autism-and-adhd-rates/
6. http://www.integrativepediatricsonline.com/blog/2013/0 4/08/genetics-and-psychiatrydisorders/
7. http://www.integrativepediatricsonline.com/blog/2013/0 4/16/depression/
8. http://www.ncbi.nlm.nih.gov/pubmed/24047633
9. http://www.ncbi.nlm.nih.gov/pubmed/15084139
10. http://www.ncbi.nlm.nih.gov/pubmed/16760626
11. http://www.ncbi.nlm.nih.gov/pubmed/22972022
12. http://www.ncbi.nlm.nih.gov/pubmed/23637840
13. http://www.ncbi.nlm.nih.gov/pubmed/23863634

Health Fitness and Wellness

1. http://www.integrativepediatricsonline.com/blog/2013/0 6/21/understanding-the-politics-of-food/
2. http://www.whilesciencesleeps.com
3. http://www.eatdrinkpolitics.com
4. http://www.ewg.org
5. http://responsibletechnology.org/media/docs/IRT_sg.p df
6. http://www.foodrevolution.org/blog/former-pro-gmo-scientist/
7. http://www.integrativepediatricsonline.com/blog/2013/0 1/18/are-you-getting-enough-sleep/
8. http://www.ncbi.nlm.nih.gov/pubmed/22946959

Diet

1. http://www.integrativepediatricsonline.com/blog/2013/07/29/vitamin-b-12-ways-to-tell-if-you-need-more-testing-for-deficiency-what-is-normal/
2. http://www.gaps.me
3. http://www.integrativepediatricsonline.com/blog/2013/04/25/you-are-what-you-eat-a-must-read/
4. http://www.integrativepediatricsonline.com/blog/2013/07/19/genetically-modified-wheat-banned-found-in-oregon-2/
5. http://www.integrativepediatricsonline.com/blog/2013/07/10/key-dos-and-donts-of-the-scd-specific-carbohydrate-or-gaps-gut-psychology-syndrome-diet/
6. http://www.integrativepediatricsonline.com/blog/2013/08/28/gmo-wheat-from-australia-presents-new-dangers/
7. http://www.integrativepediatricsonline.com/blog/2013/07/04/gmos-profit-from-poison-the-dangers-of-genetically-modified-food/
8. http://www.integrativepediatricsonline.com/blog/2013/04/04/getting-the-necessary-nutrition-from-a-vegetarian-lifestyle/
9. http://www.integrativepediatricsonline.com/blog/2013/03/20/aspartame-deadly-sweet-part-3/
10. http://www.integrativepediatricsonline.com/blog/2013/03/08/high-fructose-corn-syrup-hfcs/

11. http://www.ucdmc.ucdavis.edu/ctsc/documents/CTSC
Newsletter_Spring_2012.pdf
12. http://www.integrativepediatricsonline.com/blog/2013/
03/04/the-mediterranean-diet/
13. http://www.nejm.org/doi/full/10.1056/NEJMoa120030
3?query=OF&
14. http://www.usbiotek.com

15. http://www.integrativepediatricsonline.com/blog/2013/
02/05/toxin-methanol-foods-to-avoid/
16. http://seedsofdeception.com
17. http://www.ncbi.nlm.nih.gov/pubmed/20424937
18. http://www.ncbi.nlm.nih.gov/pubmed/20356431
19. http://www.ncbi.nlm.nih.gov/pubmed/17066209
20. http://www.ncbi.nlm.nih.gov/pubmed/17066210

Vitamins & Supplements

1. http://www.integrativepediatricsonline.com/blog/2013/08/12/conditions-that-are-often-b-12-deficiency-but-go-undetected/
2. http://www.integrativepediatricsonline.com/blog/2013/07/29/vitamin-b-12-ways-to-tell-if-you-need-more-testing-for-deficiency-what-is-normal/
3. http://www.integrativepediatricsonline.com/blog/2013/07/15/b-12-deficiency-how-common-is-it-why-is-it-missed-2/
4. http://www.ars.usda.gov/is/pr/2000/000802.htm
5. http://www.integrativepediatricsonline.com/blog/2013/06/12/vitamin-b-12-what-is-it-and-why-is-it-so-important/
6. http://www.integrativepediatricsonline.com/blog/2013/04/25/do-your-prescriptions-deplete-your-nutrients/
7. http://www.spectracell.com/clinicians/products/micronutrient-testing-comprehensive-nutritional-panel/
8. http://www.integrativepediatricsonline.com/blog/2013/07/01/any-brain-related-symptom-think-something-is-wrong-in-your-gi-track-gut-brain-connection/
9. http://www.integrativepediatricsonline.com/blog/2013/08/26/could-it-be-b-12-deficiency/
10. http://www.integrativepediatricsonline.com/blog/2013/08/07/vitamin-c-deficiencies-during-pregnancy-2/

11. http://www.integrativepediatricsonline.com/blog/2013/07/24/why-you-should-be-taking-vitamin-b-12/
12. http://www.integrativepediatricsonline.com/blog/2013/07/03/hfcs-high-fructose-corn-syrup-hidden-sources/
13. http://www.citizens.org/ten-food-items-you-might-be-surprised-to-learn-contain-hfcs-2/
14. http://www.integrativepediatricsonline.com/blog/2013/04/23/gmo-soy-experience-in-argentina-should-prompt-everyone-to-call-for-a-ban-on-gmo-foods-and-a-boycott-of-monsanto/
15. http://www.integrativepediatricsonline.com/blog/2013/04/19/top-10-food-additives-to-avoid/
16. http://www.integrativepediatricsonline.com/blog/2013/03/28/probiotics-reduce-diarrhea-allergies-asthma-and-eczema/
17. http://foodidentitytheft.com/2013/02/
18. http://www.consumerreports.org/cro/magazine/2012/11/arsenic-in-your-food/index.htm
19. "Vitamin K2 and the Calcium Paradox, How a Little Known Vitamin Could Save Your Life". By Dr.Kate Rheaume-Bleue, BSc.ND. Mississauga, Ontario: John Wiley and Sons Canada Ltd. 2012.
20. http://www.ncbi.nlm.nih.gov/pubmed/23988889
21. http://www.ncbi.nlm.nih.gov/pubmed/8698541
22. http://www.ncbi.nlm.nih.gov/pubmed/19032072
23. http://www.aacc.org/publications/cln/2011/january/Pages/folatemetabolismFigure.aspx
24. http://www.ncbi.nlm.nih.gov/pubmed/11787236
25. http://www.ncbi.nlm.nih.gov/pubmed/23449881

Exercise

1.http://www.ncbi.nlm.nih.gov/pubmed/23950908
2.http://www.ncbi.nlm.nih.gov/pubmed/18454136
3.http://www.ncbi.nlm.nih.gov/pubmed/7740249
4.http://www.ncbi.nlm.nih.gov/pubmed/23825961
5.http://www.ncbi.nlm.nih.gov/pubmed/22807642
6.http://www.ncbi.nlm.nih.gov/pubmed/11208241
7.http://www.ncbi.nlm.nih.gov/pubmed/19069254

Testing for Toxins

1. http://www.ncbi.nlm.nih.gov/pubmed/22274617
2. http://www.ehjournal.net/content/12/1/33/abstract
3. http://greenerpenny.blogspot.com/2010/01/avoiding-pbdes-in-mattresses.html
4. http://www.integrativepediatricsonline.com/blog/2013/07/12/epigenetics-dna-methylation-and-arsenic/
5. http://ehp.niehs.nih.gov/1205925/
6. http://www.integrativepediatricsonline.com/blog/2013/05/17/summary-of-plastics-which-to-avoid/
7. http://ecologycenter.org/factsheets/eliminate-plastic.pdf
8. http://www.integrativepediatricsonline.com/blog/2013/04/30/pops/
9. http://www.integrativepediatricsonline.com/blog/2013/04/17/household-cleaners-how-to-find-the-safe-ones/
10. http://www.integrativepediatricsonline.com/blog/2013/04/05/environmental-toxins/
11. http://yosemite.epa.gov/opa/admpress.nsf/0/22372FBE760C424085257B0F00686B31
12. http://www.integrativepediatricsonline.com/blog/2013/03/06/epigenetics/
13. http://www.scirp.org/journal/PaperInformation.aspx?PaperID=25083
14. http://www.integrativepediatricsonline.com/blog/2013/02/04/toxins-in-our-plastics/

15. http://www.environmentalhealthnews.org/ehs/news/2012/epa-low-dose#documentContent
16. http://www.environmentalhealthnews.org/ehs/news/2013/unep-mercury-timetoact.pdf
17. http://www.sciencedirect.com/science/article/pii/S0013935112002885
18. http://www.ewg.org
19. http://www.usbiotek.com/Services_Environmental-Pollutants-Panel.php

Bioidentical Hormones

1.http://www.ncbi.nlm.nih.gov/pubmed/19179815
2.http://www.ncbi.nlm.nih.gov/pubmed/11392031
3.http://www.ncbi.nlm.nih.gov/pubmed/?term=J+womens+hea
    lth+2000+may+9+(4)%3A+381-7
4.http://www.ncbi.nlm.nih.gov/pubmed/?term=apgar+using+pr
    ogestins+in+clinical+practice
5.http://www.ncbi.nlm.nih.gov/pubmed/?term=J+am+coll+card
    io+2000+Dec%3B36(7)%3A2154-9
6.http://www.ncbi.nlm.nih.gov/pubmed/?term=Proc+Natl+acad
    +sci+usa+2003+sep+2%3B100(18)%3A10506-11
7.http://www.ncbi.nlm.nih.gov/pubmed/?term=fertility+and+ste
    rility+journal+vol+72+issue+3+p389-397
8.http://www.ncbi.nlm.nih.gov/pubmed/?term=BJOG+oct+200
    5+vol+112+pp+1402-06

Addiction & Hormones
1.http://www.integrativepediatricsonline.com/blog/2013/0
    8/09/first-week-important-when-quitting-smoking/
2.http://www.integrativepediatricsonline.com/blog/2013/0
    7/26/cannabis-and-psychosis/
3.http://www.integrativepediatricsonline.com/blog/2013/0
    6/11/h-a-l-t/
4.http://www.ncbi.nlm.nih.gov/pubmed/23326276
5.http://www.ncbi.nlm.nih.gov/pubmed/11794469
6.http://www.aa.org
7.http://www.asam.org
8.http://www.ncbi.nlm.nih.gov/pubmed/22201971
9.http://www.ncbi.nlm.nih.gov/pubmed/19903933
10.http://www.ncbi.nlm.nih.gov/pubmed/20648912

Healthy Aging & Hormones

1. http://www.integrativepediatricsonline.com/blog/2013/0
   5/02/estrogen-mimicking-chemicals-strongly-
   distort-hormone-action/
2. http://www.integrativepediatricsonline.com/blog/2013/0
   3/26/un-who-panel-calls-hormone-disrupting-
   chemicals-a-global-threat/
3. http://www.environmentalhealthnews.org/ehs/news/20
   13/who-report
4. http://www.integrativepediatricsonline.com/blog/2013/0
   1/28/heavy-metal-toxins/
5. http://www.ncbi.nlm.nih.gov/pubmed/11836290
6. http://www.ncbi.nlm.nih.gov/pubmed/?term=2.%09Cherrier+
   MM+et+al."Testosterone+supplementation+improves+
   spatial+and+verbal+memory+in+healthy+older+men."
   +Neurology+2001%3B+57(1)%3A+80-88.
7. http://www.ncbi.nlm.nih.gov/pubmed/21693502

Hypothalamic-Pituitary Axis

1. http://www.integrativepediatricsonline.com/blog/2013/0
   8/22/lead-may-be-suppressing-the-hypothalamic-
   pituitary-axis/
2. http://ehp.niehs.nih.gov/1206105/
3. http://www.ehjournal.net/content/12/1/26
4. http://www.ncbi.nlm.nih.gov/pubmed/17106184
5. http://www.ncbi.nlm.nih.gov/pubmed/23530988

Thyroid

1. http://ehp.niehs.nih.gov/1205092/
2. http://www.ncbi.nlm.nih.gov/pubmed/23781319
3. http://www.ncbi.nlm.nih.gov/pmc/articles/PMC3613903
4. http://www.ncbi.nlm.nih.gov/pubmed/?term=J+clin+endocrin
    ology+Metab+2005+May%3B+90(5)%3A2666-74
5. http://www.ncbi.nlm.nih.gov/pubmed/?term=biol+trace+elem
    +res+1996+Jan%3B+51(1)%3A31-41
6. http://www.ncbi.nlm.nih.gov/pubmed/9971866
7. http://www.ncbi.nlm.nih.gov/pubmed/10681281
8. http://www.ncbi.nlm.nih.gov/pubmed/?term=JAMA+dec+1+2
    004%2C+vol+292+thyroid+status+in+old+age
9. http://www.ncbi.nlm.nih.gov/pubmed/?term=preventive+card
    iology+2001++an+association+between+varying+degr
    ess+of+hypothyroidism+and+hypercholesterolemia+in
    +women%3A+the+thyroid-cholesterol+connection
10. http://www.ncbi.nlm.nih.gov/pubmed/?term=jcem+vol+92+
    no+5+1715-1723
11. http://www.ncbi.nlm.nih.gov/pubmed/23843809

DHEA/Steroid Hormones

1.http://www.ncbi.nlm.nih.gov/pubmed/24047936
2.http://www.ncbi.nlm.nih.gov/pubmed/21586137
3.http://www.ncbi.nlm.nih.gov/pubmed/23824417
4.http://www.ncbi.nlm.nih.gov/pubmed/23737215
5.http://www.ncbi.nlm.nih.gov/pubmed/23664458
6.http://www.ncbi.nlm.nih.gov/pubmed/23647054
7.http://www.ncbi.nlm.nih.gov/pubmed/14551720
8.http://www.ncbi.nlm.nih.gov/pubmed/15783247
9.http://www.ncbi.nlm.nih.gov/pubmed/11109974
10.http://www.ncbi.nlm.nih.gov/pubmed/21976778
11.http://www.ncbi.nlm.nih.gov/pubmed/20610590

Testosterone for Men

1.http://www.ncbi.nlm.nih.gov/pubmed/16760626
2.http://www.ncbi.nlm.nih.gov/pubmed/15084139
3.http://www.ncbi.nlm.nih.gov/pubmed/24047633
4.http://www.ncbi.nlm.nih.gov/pubmed/23219010
5.http://www.ncbi.nlm.nih.gov/pmc/articles/PMC1472881
6.http://www.ncbi.nlm.nih.gov/pubmed/19440073
7.http://www.ncbi.nlm.nih.gov/pubmed/21982312
8.http://www.ncbi.nlm.nih.gov/pubmed/21976718
9.http://www.ncbi.nlm.nih.gov/pubmed/22777902
10.http://www.ncbi.nlm.nih.gov/pubmed/18413429
11.http://www.ncbi.nlm.nih.gov/pubmed/18230794
12.http://www.ncbi.nlm.nih.gov/pubmed/17911176
13.http://www.ncbi.nlm.nih.gov/pubmed/17060543
14.http://www.ncbi.nlm.nih.gov/pubmed/10523014
15.http://www.ncbi.nlm.nih.gov/pubmed/10022418
16.http://www.ncbi.nlm.nih.gov/pubmed/1547923
17.http://www.ncbi.nlm.nih.gov/pubmed/?term=3.%09Ch
    errier+MM+et+al."Cognitive+effects+of+short-
    term+manipulation+of+serum+sex+steroids+in+h
    ealthy+young+men."+J+Clin+Endocrinol+Metab+
    2002%3B+87(7)%3A+3%2C090-3%2C096.
18.http://www.ncbi.nlm.nih.gov/pubmed/?term=4.%09Ch
    errier+MM%2C+Craft+S%2C+Matsumoto+AH."C
    ognitive+changes+associated+with+supplementat
    ion+of+testosterone+or+dihydrotestosterone+in+
    mildly+hypogonadal+men%3A+a+preliminary+rep
    ort."+J+Androl+2003%3B+24(4)%3A+568-576.

Testosterone for Women

1. http://www.ncbi.nlm.nih.gov/pubmed/12945798
2. http://www.ncbi.nlm.nih.gov/pubmed/22449989
3. http://www.ncbi.nlm.nih.gov/pubmed/11304876
4. http://www.ncbi.nlm.nih.gov/pubmed/23627249
5. http://www.ncbi.nlm.nih.gov/pubmed/23912530
6. http://www.ncbi.nlm.nih.gov/pubmed/23352690
7. http://www.ncbi.nlm.nih.gov/pubmed/10573435

Estrogen/progesterone (women)

1. http://www.integrativepediatricsonline.com/blog/2013/0 5/01/memory-and-cognitive-function/
2. http://www.ncbi.nlm.nih.gov/pubmed/23627249
3. http://www.ncbi.nlm.nih.gov/pubmed/23969765
4. http://www.ncbi.nlm.nih.gov/pubmed/9409295
5. http://www.ncbi.nlm.nih.gov/pubmed/17217322
6. http://www.ncbi.nlm.nih.gov/pubmed/15111738
7. http://www.ncbi.nlm.nih.gov/pubmed/15883113
8. http://www.ncbi.nlm.nih.gov/pmc/articles/PMC3042920/?rep ort=reader
9. http://www.ncbi.nlm.nih.gov/pubmed/17217322
10. http://www.ncbi.nlm.nih.gov/pubmed/10519605
11. http://www.ncbi.nlm.nih.gov/pubmed/10868610
12. http://www.ncbi.nlm.nih.gov/pubmed/9743505
13. http://www.ncbi.nlm.nih.gov/pubmed/?term=circulatio n+1999%3B+100%3A+2319
14. http://www.ncbi.nlm.nih.gov/pubmed/21489728
15. http://www.ncbi.nlm.nih.gov/pubmed/12627037

Melatonin

1. http://www.ncbi.nlm.nih.gov/pubmed/24051052
2. http://www.ncbi.nlm.nih.gov/pubmed/24033914
3. http://www.ncbi.nlm.nih.gov/pubmed/24032643
4. http://www.ncbi.nlm.nih.gov/pmc/articles/PMC3051850
   /
5. http://www.ncbi.nlm.nih.gov/pubmed/23853635

Vitamin D

1. http://www.integrativepediatricsonline.com/blog/2013/0 9/18/why-you-need-vitamin-k-2-and-how-it-interacts-with-calcium-and-vitamin-d/
2. http://www.integrativepediatricsonline.com/blog/2013/0 9/10/calcium-vitamin-d-and-obesity/
3. http://www.ncbi.nlm.nih.gov/pubmed/15879568
4. http://www.integrativepediatricsonline.com/blog/2013/0 9/03/vitamin-d-deficiency-leading-to-rapidly-aging-bones-and-fractures/
5. http://quintaisimortais.blogspot.com/2013/07/vitamin-d-deficiency-linked-to.html
6. http://ods.od.nih.gov/factsheets/VitaminD-HealthProfessional/
7. http://www.integrativepediatricsonline.com/blog/2013/0 8/27/how-much-vitamin-d-can-i-get-from-my-diet-fish-milk-fortified-cereals/
8. http://www.integrativepediatricsonline.com/blog/2013/0 8/06/vitamin-d-and-your-brain-more-than-an-antidepressant-and-can-affect-your-unborn-childs-brain/
9. http://www.vitamindcouncil.org/newsletter/newsletter-pregnancy-and-gestational-vitamin-d-deficiency/
10. http://www.integrativepediatricsonline.com/blog/2013/ 07/30/vitamin-d-deficiency-who-is-affected-and-at-the-highest-risk/
11. http://archinte.jamanetwork.com/article.aspx?articleid =414878

12. http://www.integrativepediatricsonline.com/blog/2013/ 06/25/vitamin-d-what-is-it-what-are-its-main- functions/
13. http://www.integrativepediatricsonline.com/blog/2013/ 09/17/vitamin-d-toxicity-when-you-take-too-much- vitamin-d/
14. http://www.mayoclinic.com/health/vitamin-d- toxicity/AN02008
15. http://www.ncbi.nlm.nih.gov/pubmed/22274617
16. http://www.integrativepediatricsonline.com/blog/2013/ 07/16/is-your-vit-d-supplement-reliable-jama- article/
17. http://archinte.jamanetwork.com/article.aspx?articleid =1570096
18. http://www.integrativepediatricsonline.com/blog/2013/ 05/06/vitamin-d-and-gut-flora/
19. http://www.journals.elsevierhealth.com/periodicals/ajp a/article/S0002-9440(10)60126-5/abstract
20. http://www.ncbi.nlm.nih.gov/pubmed/23922354
21. http://www.grassrootshealth.net/media/download/dip_ with_numbers_8-24-12.pdf

Growth Hormone

1.http://www.ncbi.nlm.nih.gov/pubmed/6345147
    2.http://www.ncbi.nlm.nih.gov/pubmed/10905377
3.http://www.ncbi.nlm.nih.gov/pubmed/24019611

Goals/ lab values

1http://www.spectracell.com/media/uploaded/2/0e20081
    45_252fullpaper1993acla-functional-analytical-
    technique-for-monitoring-nutrient-status--part-
    3.pdf
2.http://www.spectracell.com/media/uploaded/2/0e20081
    71_251fullpaper1993acla-functional-analytical-
    technique-for-monitoring-nutrient-status--part-
    2.pdf
3.http://www.spectracell.com/media/uploaded/1/0e20081
    07_187fullpaper2004janahpas-study.pdf
4.http://www.spectracell.com/media/uploaded/1/0e20081
    15_186fullpaper2001janafiaofnutritionalandantioxi
    dantstatus.pdf
5.http://www.ncbi.nlm.nih.gov/pubmed/20400494

www.ingramcontent.com/pod-product-compliance
Lightning Source LLC
Chambersburg PA
CBHW071057290526
45795CB00004B/1543